# Shiny Hair

## *Simple and Effective Ways to Get Strong, Shiny, Healthy, Sexy Hair*

by Luna Hirsch

# Table of Contents

Introduction.........................................................................1

Chapter 1: A Nutrient Rich Diet....................................5

Chapter 2: Choosing the Right Shampoo and Hair
Conditioner.................................................................13

Chapter 3: Preventing Hair Damage When Styling...17

Chapter 4: Give Yourself a Regular Scalp Massage ..21

Chapter 5: Hot or Cold Water: Which Is the Best? ..23

Chapter 6: Wet Hair Restrictions .................................27

Chapter 7: Choose the Right Hair Brush....................31

Chapter 8: Hair Serum Magic .......................................35

Chapter 9: Removing Hair Product Buildup on Hair
.................................................................................39

Chapter 10: Protecting Hair from the Effects of
Chlorine.........................................................................43

Chapter 11: Trying Out Homemade Hair Treatments ..................................................................47

Chapter 12: Asking the Experts ....................................51

Chapter 13: Proper Hygiene ..........................................55

Conclusion ........................................................................57

# Introduction

Hair is a major component of your physical appearance that is immediately noticed, whether consciously or subconsciously, every time you see or interact with other people. Believe it or not, hair actually affects your overall appeal and attractiveness, which is one of many reasons why people try so hard to take good care of their hair. Shiny and healthy hair helps you make a good impression, so why not take action so as to improve its appearance?

Read on now to discover all the effective ways to get shiny, strong, healthy, and sexy hair!

# Chapter 1: A Nutrient Rich Diet

Having a healthy diet improves your overall health. And this includes the health of your hair. Your scalp contains cells, and several processes take place in that area of your body. For all of these to be fully functional, it must obtain the right amount of vitamins and nutrients. It may not seem as if your hair is being affected by what you eat. But it actually is. Unlike your skin, it will take time for your hair to display either the positive or the negative effects of your existing diet, because it needs time to grow.

The follicles of your hair are fortified with the nutrients that your body gets. By having a healthy and balanced diet, you will get to have healthier hair follicles and a healthier scalp. Consequently, you will enjoy healthier and more beautiful hair. It's not just a proper diet that affects the condition of your hair. There are several other elements that you have to factor in. Provided below are some of the most efficient food items that can help you improve your hair's health.

## A. Protein Rich Foods

Remember that your hair is composed of around 97% protein. It only makes sense for you to supply an ample amount of this kind of nutrient to your hair. What better way to do this than to eat foods that are rich in protein. Your hair needs protein so that it'll be nice and strong. Every day, strands of your hair fall out. If you do not include sufficient amount of protein in your diet, your body will not be capable of creating new hair to replace the ones that you have lost.

Also, your hair is made of keratin which is a specific type of protein. It plays a very important role in keeping your hair strong and elastic. If you do not eat foods that are rich in protein, you will be putting your hair at risk of easy damage and breakage. Also, this can cause thinning hair because lesser protein intake will force your hair to lose its pigmentation.

You can enjoy eating turkey, chicken, lamb, beef, pork, and fish. You can also indulge yourself in eating yogurt, eggs and various dairy products. Just make sure that you eat all these in moderation, especially if you do not want to gain weight.

## B. Foods High in Omega 3 Fatty Acids

Aside from protein, your hair is composed of 3% fat. This particular percentage of fat is responsible for producing oil within your scalp. They are very important because they keep your hair and scalp from drying out. Drying of the scalp and hair can cause several problems such as dandruff. It may even cause your hair to turn brittle and dry. In order to avoid this, you need to include foods rich in omega 3 fatty acids in your diet.

Salmon is the best example of a food type that is rich in Omega 3 fatty acids. It is also packed with vitamin D and both of these are responsible for keeping your hair strong and healthy. If in case you are not fond of eating salmon, you can try out other food types that are full of this kind of nutrient. These include mackerel, trout, walnuts, avocado, flax seed, and whole grain products.

## C. Vitamin A, B Complex, C, and E Rich Foods

It is also highly recommended for you to eat foods that are rich in vitamin A. It will help you maintain the health of your scalp by protecting the oil that it contains. Vitamin A along with its anti-oxidants are responsible for moisturizing your hair and your scalp thus, preventing it from drying. It is also responsible for the growth, thickness and darkness of your hair.

In addition to that, since Vitamin A contains anti-oxidants, it can protect your hair from the harmful damages that might be caused by free radicals. Consequently, the natural shine of your hair will be restored and exposed. Vitamin A also contains properties that can repair and regenerate your hair. It will help your hair become smooth and soft. Food items that are rich in Vitamin A include sweet potatoes, yogurt, oysters, tomatoes and carrots.

Vitamin B Complex helps in preventing your hair from becoming brittle and weak. It is also responsible for giving you that gorgeous rich hair color through its melanin component. Also, Biotin, which is a part of the vitamin B family, can help improve the texture of your hair. With a sufficient amount of biotin included in your diet, that'll help in increasing your hair's growth rate, improve the thickness of your hair and make it a lot stronger. Some of the foods that are rich in biotin include cauliflower, raspberries, eggs and bananas.

To prevent hair loss, it is also a must to eat foods that are rich in Vitamin B12. Hair loss is commonly attributed to your body's lack of Iron. By taking more vitamin B12, you will get to improve your body's absorption of Iron which will then lead to the prevention of hair loss. Some of the foods abundant in Vitamin B12 include cheese, yogurt, egg and milk.

Nobody wants to have gray hair simply because it is the most visible sign of aging. There are a lot of people who experience premature graying of their hair at a very young age. By eating foods that are filled with vitamin c, you will not only prevent your hair from turning gray, but you will also prevent it from drying out. Aside from taking in vitamin c supplements, you can also eat strawberries, mandarin, lemons and guava as they are the best source of this kind of vitamin.

Hair growth is also promoted by vitamin E and that is why you have to include almonds, fish, milk and peanuts in your diet. Also, vitamin E has been proven to fight off various kinds of hair problems such as drying and roughness. It prevents moisture from leaving, thus helping your hair to retain its natural shine.

## D. Iron and Zinc

Eating foods rich in Iron and Zinc are also important in maintaining the health and natural shine of your hair. Iron promotes the circulation of oxygen to the follicles of your hair. It prevents hair loss. Several studies have been conducted and their researches have proven that lack of iron leads to baldness. In order to avoid this dilemma which will potentially hamper the quality of your life and not to mention your overall appeal, you should include foods such as lean beef, oysters, lamb, chicken and pork to your diet. These food types are all rich in Iron including eggs, soybeans and even brown rice.

Also, to avoid dryness of hair and scalp and hair loss, you also have to include foods rich in zinc to your diet. It promotes hair strengthening and it also encourages the growth of long and beautiful hair. Some of the foods rich in zinc include yogurt, beef, eggs and lamb.

# Chapter 2: Choosing the Right Shampoo and Hair Conditioner

Even if you are eating a healthy diet but you are using the incorrect type of shampoo and conditioner for your hair, then you may just end up doing more damage to your hair. It is a must to choose the right type of shampoo and conditioner to ensure that your hair is not only clean but healthy and strong at the same time.

## A. Choosing a Shampoo

Before you purchase any kind of shampoo regardless of its brand, you need to know what it can do and how to use it. It must also be appropriate for your hair and scalp type. If you have dry hair or scalp, then you have to choose a shampoo that will help moisturize it and bring back its natural texture. You should also choose one that does not contain any ingredient that may lead to hair damage. Avoid brands that have sulfates, silicon and those that have a high concentration of alcohol. Using a shampoo with these damaging ingredients will eliminate the natural oils found in your hair and eventually damage it with prolonged use.

If you are having problems with frizzy hair, then it would be best to choose a shampoo that is anti-frizz. Also, if you are having problems with dandruff, then you have to specifically choose shampoos that are created to help in removing dandruff.

## B. Choosing a Conditioner

When it comes to choosing the right type of conditioner, the process may be quite overwhelming if you do not know what you are looking for. There are several brands out there promising you to have shiny, beautiful and healthy hair but not all of them actually work. Conditioners are designed to replace the moisture that has been lost when you shampooed your hair. It has the ability to smoothen your hair cuticle and levels your hair pH. Conditioners will also help you untangle and promote much more manageable hair.

If you have an oily scalp, you may consider avoiding conditioners that are meant to moisturize or hydrate. You must choose those that will add volume to your hair and help strengthen it instead. If you have dry and brittle hair, then you have to avoid conditioners that are designed to increase hair volume. You have to choose those that are meant to moisturize and hydrate instead. You should also look for a conditioner that is meant to repair hair damage and promotes frizz control.

# Chapter 3: Preventing Hair Damage When Styling

You may be one of the many people who love to use a flat or curling iron when styling your hair. Though these tools may help you achieve the hair style and the look that you're going for, they can also lead to hair damage. These devices can reach up to 400 degrees of heat temperature! This will undoubtedly cause damage to your hair, especially if you are styling wet or unprotected hair. You may not see its effects immediately, but in the long run you will end up with some serious split ends and your hair will be more prone to breakage.

You can prevent this from happening without having to stop styling your hair by using certain products that can help protect your hair during styling. There are a lot of products that prevent overheating topically. Here are some steps that you can follow.

- You need to make sure that your hair is completely dry before you style it using your flat or curling iron. The chemical composition of your hair is altered if heat is applied on wet hair. In addition to that, it can also damage your hair and it may also lead to dandruff.

- Make sure that you use effective "heat protection" styling products before you reshape your hair. These kinds of products will help protect your hair from the heat. You can choose from the many options available in the market.

- Apply these heat protection products when your hair is still wet, but then wait for your hair to dry before styling.

- Use styling devices that have ceramic surfaces because the metal ones can damage your hair.

# Chapter 4: Give Yourself a Regular Scalp Massage

Having healthy hair means having a healthy scalp. And in order to have that, you will need to stimulate your scalp to prevent potential problems from occurring. You can do this by massaging your scalp. It does not only promote better mental function, but it also aids in giving you healthier hair. It keeps your hair in better shape and it improves circulation of oxygen and nutrients in your scalp. This is a routine that is fairly easy. There are several ways to do this.

The first and the simplest way of massaging your scalp is with the use of your hands. No devices required because all you need are your fingers. Make sure that you are comfortably seated without any distractions. Place your fingers on your forehead and gently apply pressure then release. Work your way up to your hairline the reapply pressure and then release. Repeat this procedure up until you reach your scalp. Once done, move your way down to the back of your scalp and continue gently with the pressure and release movement. Once you have reached your nape, you can now go back towards your forehead using the same movements.

# Chapter 5: Hot or Cold Water: Which Is the Best?

Normally, you will simply get in the shower and blast your hair with hot water. That is the typical routine of many people. However, several studies have shown that using cold or hot water has effects on the health of your hair. Provided below are some points for you to consider if you are truly serious in having shiny and healthy hair.

Let us first consider the use of hot water. It has its own pros and cons. The best thing about hot water is that it helps remove the dirt and excess oil in your hair as you take a shower. Hot water will open your pores which will then promote the process of exfoliation and removal of excess oils. If you are one of the many people who have oily scalps, then using hot water can be very helpful. It also allows dirt to be removed from the pores of your scalp.

However, using hot water too often can result to having overly porous hair. This will eventually lead to having dry and brittle hair. These are the disadvantages of using hot water all the time. It can either make or break the health of your hair. Although it washes away the dirt out of your hair, it can also remove your hair's natural oils which are responsible for making it shine naturally. Hot water can cause your hair to lose its moisture, which will then lead to having a frizzy and unmanageable hair.

What about cold water? It actually works in opposite with hot water. Cold water causes your pores to close. Because of this, dirt will be prevented from entering your scalp, thus, avoiding its accumulation. It also seals in the moisture in your hair cuticle and this can be very beneficial, especially if you have just applied conditioner. This prevents your hair from becoming dry and frizzy. Cold water also promotes the natural shine of your hair. That is one reason why several stylists chose to blast cold air after they blow dry. This same concept is applicable to using cold water when rinsing your hair. It adds luster and smoothness to your hair.

Use all of the above knowledge to customize your shower experience based on the current status of your hair. And when all else fails, wash with hot water, then at the very end just before turning off the water, turn the lever to the cold setting, and painfully stick your head under until the hair has been fully doused with cold water to close off the pores. Your hair will definitely be shinier that day for doing so.

# Chapter 6: Wet Hair Restrictions

It is also important for you to remember that brushing wet hair is not advisable. This is because you can easily damage your hair when it this state. Wet hair is more delicate when compared to dry hair, especially when it comes to brushing. It is in a vulnerable state because the hydrogen bonds in your hair have been broken after showering. Instead of using a brush, it's best to use a wide tooth comb or a bristled brush. If you use these instead of a brush, you will lessen hair breakage in the middle.

Also, while tying or wrapping your hair tightly can make you look good, this will potentially damage your hair if you do it while your hair is still wet. You have to remember that your hair may potentially be damaged, especially when it is wet. If you tie your wet hair, you are encouraging the weakening of your hair strands. When this happens, and if you do this all the time, you will begin to come across several hair problems.

You will probably be shedding more hair every time your hair is wet. If you tie it, it will not only weaken your hair, but it will also be prone to breakage. This will eventually lead to hair damage. In order to avoid this, you have to be patient in gently drying your hair with the use of a soft towel.

Tying your hair when it is wet can also cause hair loss, dandruff and itchy scalp. If you have dandruff, of course you can expect that you will have an itchy scalp. These happen because sweat and moisture are trapped whenever you tie your wet hair. You can avoid this by making sure that your hair is completely dry.

# Chapter 7: Choose the Right Hair Brush

Choosing the right hair brush is also very important in maintaining the health of your hair. Your hair brush goes beyond the mere function of helping you style your hair. It plays a role in massaging your scalp too. It can even help in cleaning your hair follicles and remove dirt on your scalp. It helps stimulate the production and release of natural oils that will make your hair shine. In order to enjoy these benefits, you need to make sure that you choose the right kind of brush. There are several types available in the market today and choosing one can be confusing. Here are some tips that you can follow.

Use a boar bristle brush for your daily brushing. You can use this to follow the old saying "100 strokes a day for a beautiful hair". Make sure that the bristles are made from nylon. The combination of the boar and these bristles will help you have perfectly polished hair.

You also need to use a natural boar bristle brush when blow drying and straightening your hair. You do not have to exert that much effort because this kind of brush will help smooth and lengthen your hair.

If you have thick hair and want to style it flatter, then use a paddle shaped brush. On the other hand, if you want your hair to have that much loved sexy volume, you need to use round hair brushes. It adds curls and it is very helpful when it comes to hair styling. For removing hair tangles, it is highly recommended to use square and cushioned paddle hair brushes.

Once you have found the right kind of brush, you now have to make sure that you properly brush your hair. Doing this on a regular basis helps your hair rejuvenate. This is even more effective if coupled with scalp massage.

Regular brushing encourages the removal of dirt from your hair. It also helps in removing waste materials in your scalp such as uric acid crystal deposits, catarrh and several other acids that build up in your scalp over time. The blood capillaries in your scalp are also stimulated through brushing. It helps in promoting better circulation of nutrients and oxygen to your scalp and hair. In addition to that, it helps your hair in maintaining its natural oils plus it adds luster and volume to your hair.

# Chapter 8: Hair Serum Magic

We've all been stunned by the gorgeous, shiny and beautiful hair that celebrities and models have. Also, every now and then you will get to see several ads promising to help you have that shiny and healthy hair that you have always dreamed of. However, if you are one of the millions of people who are living a hectic lifestyle, spending too much time on styling your hair is a luxury that you just cannot afford. Good thing there are products that can help you out instantly. One of these products is known as the hair serum.

This product is silicone based and it is used in coating one's hair. It is even capable of changing the structure of your hair because it can penetrate your hair's cuticles. Because of its said efficiency, several brands are now available in the market. You need to make sure that you find the best one that matches your needs and your hair type.

Hair serum helps in making your hair instantly shinier. It helps reduce hair tangles which are quite difficult to manage. It also protects your hair from the harmful effects of humidity and dust. Not only that, it can also protect your hair from sun damage and the effects of various other chemicals.

In most cases, products like these are used to prevent hair damage and dryness. There have been a lot of people who have been using it because they wish to get rid of their frizzy and tangled hair. Others use it to protect their hair from the harmful effects of regular styling.

If you are one of the many people who are planning to use this hair product, there are certain things that you have to consider. First of all, you have to choose a trusted brand. Do not solely base your decision on the price because not all are actually effective. You must also remember that you should not rub the serum to your scalp. Apply it to your hair using your fingers or by using a comb. Also, make sure that the serum that you have chosen works perfectly well with the shampoo and conditioner that you are using. Lastly, make sure that you do not overuse it because anything in excess is bad. This may lead to dandruff and other hair problems.

# Chapter 9: Removing Hair Product Buildup on Hair

If you are one of the many people who constantly use hair products, you need to also give your hair and scalp some rest and pamper them every now and then. Hair product buildup may cause your hair to be difficult to style plus it can even cause dandruff and itchiness. This is one of the countless reasons why you have to do deep cleansing. In most cases, over the counter clarifying shampoos can do the trick. However, there are instances when you will need to do something more than that.

You can also use apple cider vinegar. The process is quite simple. You just have to wash your hair thoroughly and use the apple cider vinegar on the final rinsing of your hair. It will help remove any residue in your hair. Experts also suggest alternating between high quality and low-quality hair products. High quality hair products are great for making your hair look healthy and shiny. However, it can also damage your hair. By using low quality ones that are rich in alkaline content, the buildup will be removed. However, you must only do this occasionally.

Another effective thing to use to remove the buildup is baking soda because it acts as an antacid on your hair. You can do this by creating a paste made from the combination of a few parts of baking soda and your shampoo. Use it the way you use your regular shampoo and leave it for about 5 minutes before rinsing your hair. After rinsing the paste, you can use your regular conditioner afterwards.

The best way to resolve this is to avoid the buildup. You can do this by avoiding the use of products that contain waxes and oils because they are the main cause of the buildup. It would be best if you use products that contain hydrolyzed proteins instead. Always remember that if your hair is free from any buildup, you can enjoy more naturally shiny and healthy hair.

# Chapter 10: Protecting Hair from the Effects of Chlorine

Everybody loves to go for a swim. However, chlorine can damage your hair significantly. The water in swimming pools usually contains chlorine. So, how can you enjoy your swim without having to worry about damaging your hair?

Chlorine, though effective in killing harmful bacteria in water can also remove the natural oils in your hair. These natural oils are very important because it protects your hair from daily wear and other forms of damages. It would be best to apply protective hair products before you jump into the pool such as silicon-based hair products. You can also use coconut oil to protect your hair from the damaging effects of chlorine.

You can also use swim caps to protect your hair from absorbing the chlorine content of the water in the pool. Although, it will not block the water entirely, it can help minimize its effects. It is also important to have on hand some hair cleansers which you can use when you take a shower after swimming in the pool. Remember that chlorine cannot be washed away with soap and water. You will need something stronger. There are several products available in the market that

are developed to help you remove chlorine from your
hair.

# Chapter 11: Trying Out Homemade Hair Treatments

There are several things that you can do at home that can help you have that much wanted shiny hair. There are some who are naturally gifted while most of us will have to exert some effort to achieve this goal. There are various home treatments that you can use to help you get that beautiful hair.

### A. Use Coconut Oil

This treatment will require you to use unrefined coconut oil. This is very effective especially if you have dry hair. However, if you have an oily scalp, make sure that you do not rub it too much and avoid applying it to close to your hairline. The amount that you need will depend on the thickness of your hair, but in any case, is typically much less than expected. Start from the tips and move your way up as you apply this treatment. The first time you try it, start with the amount no larger than the volume of an average peanut M&M.

## B. Vinegar

You can also use vinegar to treat your hair. This will help you restore its natural ph. It will give your hair the shine and the glow that you want to have, and this treatment is most effective if you add lemon juice to it. Use this mix as your final rinse. You will enjoy shinier and smoother hair once you are done with it.

## C. Mayonnaise

You can also use mayonnaise. This is not only good for burgers but also for your hair. It will help improve your dry hair by giving it more moisture since it can act as a hair mask. You can use regular mayonnaise and even add some vanilla extract to give it a more pleasant scent. Once done with this treatment, your hair will have the luster that you have always dreamed of.

# Chapter 12: Asking the Experts

Although there are several methods that you can do at home and by yourself that can help you take care of your hair, nothing beats the assistance obtained only from the hair experts. There are a lot of them out there offering services that will help your hair look perfect. Not only will they be treating your hair, they can also offer you some advice on how to take care of your hair properly.

When finding the right expert, make sure that you check their reputation. You can ask your family members, your friends and even your colleagues if they know someone who can give assist you with your hair problems. They will be able to give you firsthand information about the professional that they've been to especially if they used to have the same hair problems that you have now.

You can check online for the reviews of their previous customers. This will help you gauge the quality of their service. Also, do not forget to check on the various products that they are going to use if in case you opt to get their hair treatment servicers. They must be able to explain why that's their chosen product for your treatment and explain the ingredients contained in those products. This is just to avoid ending up having more hair problems instead of actually resolving those that you currently have.

# Chapter 13: Proper Hygiene

The best way to keep not only your hair but also your entire body healthy is to have proper hygiene. This is the basic and the most important aspect when it comes to your overall health and wellness. Proper hygiene includes proper hair care. This means that you have to take a bath every day. You also need to make sure that you clean and rinse your hair properly. Being always on the go does not mean that you have to let go of this practice. Even if you are busy, you need to find time to care not only for your hair but to take care of your entire body.

# Conclusion

Hair Care is very important not only because it will help you make a good impression or make you look good in front of others. Taking care of your hair will give you self-confidence and it will also boost your self-esteem. There are a lot of things that you can do so that you can enjoy having shiny, healthy, and sexy hair. I hope this book has helped inspire you to try out a few new ways to make your hair look even better than it does now. If you enjoyed this book, please leave a review on Amazon. Thank you!

Printed in Poland
by Amazon Fulfillment
Poland Sp. z o.o., Wrocław

54126227R00038